30 Essential Running Workouts, 30 Minutes or Less

Simple But Effective Running Workouts for the Busy Runner

Von Collins

Contents

Introduction

Whether you're a weekend runner, an Olympian, or simply a fitness enthusiast, you probably know about the importance of highly-efficient, time-saving workouts.

It would be great if we all had unlimited leisure time for our training, and whitespace in our schedule for fitness. The truth is that most of us have limited time. In fact, for many of us, time is the most valuable commodity in our lives.

When it comes to improving your running and overall fitness, a combination of quality and quantity is important in your training. There are some days when a nice, long run is just what the coach ordered. But there are also times when a precise, challenging, 30-minute workout is ideal for both your schedule and your training plan.

This book is intended to show you 30 great workouts that will be a perfect fit in your running training plan, and each can be done in 30 minutes or less. I know that you will not always be able to find 60 or 90 or more minutes for a workout, but you should be able to routinely find 30 minutes for a high-quality training session.

I hope you enjoy these workouts as much as I do.

A Little Background

I am dedicated to helping you be more active, and achieve your fitness goals. Whether you want to be the next Ironman competitor or do the local 5K, I try to make fitness and athletics accessible to everybody.

For an athlete, the hardest part is deciding you are going to do it, and committing to a training regimen. If you have this book, then you are already doing that!

As an avid triathlete, road runner, and coach to many aspiring racers around the USA, I love staying plugged-in to the training and racing culture. To-date, I have done 60+ triathlons and distance running races, and have been studying the topic for 27 years.

I am also obviously an author, and have been featured at Complete Tri, the NY Times, Active. USA Triathlon, Readers Digest, and many other media outlets and major organizations.

My other books include:

Your First Triathlon Guide - My top-selling book, helping people around the world enter the sport of triathlon. Find it here.

Running Smarter - 21 workout and nutrition "hacks' to help you become a more capable runner, regardless of your goals. Find it here.

Fit Foods - A guide on how athletes can use everyday nutrition to their advantage, in a way that is actionable and sustainable. Find it here.

If you want to hear about **the best running tips and gear deals I am finding**, feel free sign up for my mailing list. I only email when there is something valuable for you. Don't worry, you will never get spammed. <u>Sign up here.</u>

Philosophy

As you read through this book and select workouts to fit into your training plan, it is important to understand the philosophy behind our workouts. In short, our core philosophy can be boiled down into a few points:

- Fitness or athletic improvement is a total-body project, not something where you spot train a muscle group or lung capacity or flexibility. That's why your workouts for any given week should include a wide range of exercise types to work your entire body system, including your mental game.

- Injury prevention is paramount to a successful fitness campaign. If you're sidelined, you're not improving. While this book is not necessarily about stretching, core training, routine rehabilitation, or health maintenance, those concepts are referred to often and should be a continuous part of any training plan.

- The right balance of workout concepts should include a combination of aerobic, anaerobic, speed, duration, technique, and mental work. Taken in concert, activities from these different areas will help you improve toward your goals. Every week should

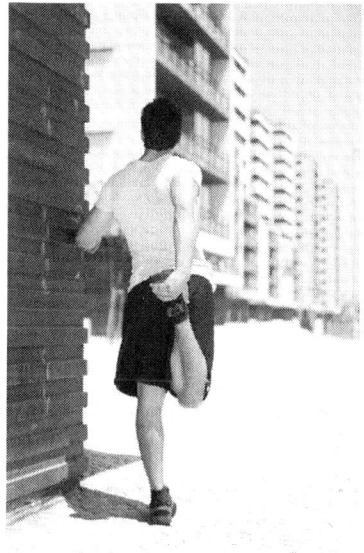

include a broad mix of these various concepts, with added emphasis on one or two based on your specific workout goals or race plans.

- Training precision is critical. Breaking out of the rut of going on the same run every day will do wonders for your fitness as well as your race times. A well-designed 30-minute workout will probably have more impact on your conditioning than a random, low-intensity longer run. Because of the need for precision, I recommend a good, basic, multisport watch to use as your training companion.

- Listen to your body. Your body will tell you if you're not ready to go at 100% on some of these workouts, or if you might be choosing an endurance distance that's a little too long for you. We recommend augmenting your body's voice with a stopwatch or pace watch (GPS-enabled) as well as a heart-rate monitor, as they can add precision and understanding to your workout.

An Important Note

Many of the workouts in this book are geared toward people who are already actively training and need some ideas on how to inject variety into their routine. As such, the intensity levels on some of these workouts can be very high.

If you are a novice or just beginning a workout plan, consider starting with a "base" period where you gradually build your cardiac output and teach your body how to function as an active system. After you complete a base period of four to eight weeks (depending on your fitness starting point), it is time to increase your intensity and endurance. Be careful to approach your training in a way that complements your total health and current fitness level.

Consider using a heart rate monitor to help you understand how your body is responding to various exertion levels. If you are brand new to working out, consult a physician first to be sure that your body is prepared for a workout routine.

Additionally, I do not explicitly build stretching in to each 30 minute running workout I describe, but you need to stretch. Do it both before and after your workout, and if you are due for an intense workout or are feeling tight, consider adding a brief stretch at the conclusion of your 7-minute warm-up.

Why the 7 - minute warmup?

You will quickly notice that for each of these 30-minute training sessions, I recommend a 7-minute warmup. In some cases, it might be six minutes, if the first phase of the workout is relatively lite.

Why seven minutes? What is magical about that duration?

I should note that the perfect warmup length is different for everyone. The only scientific way to find out what is right for you is to take a VO2 Max test. This is that test that you see people at your health club take, with a mask over their face. Among other things, it measures your output and oxygen consumption at various levels, and will help you understand at what point your lungs and muscles are adequately warmed-up for more intensity.

For most runners in decent shape, that point comes between the 5 and 10 minute mark of exertion. 7 minutes is the zone where I observe that many runners have gradually increased their heart rate, and adequately loosened-up muscles and allowed all muscle groups to participate in the movement. Your warmup will also allow your body to get into its efficient and healthy running gait. Believe it or not, when you first start running, your joint alignment and running motion can be off, even though you do it all the time. After 5-7 minutes, most runners have achieved good alignment, cadence, and stride.

A good warmup is done at a conversation pace, progressively faster with each minute, but never to a point of significant exertion. I write more about the importance of a good warmup in _Running Smarter._

Section 1:
Road Running Workouts

For any runner, running workouts are obviously the core part of your training plan, and for most runners, road running (which also includes paved and even trail running) is the most accessible form of a running workout. Usually, these runs can be done from your front door!

First, I will focus on a few of the iconic run workouts that every runner needs to know, and do. Then, I will go in to some of the variations or riffs on these runs that can give your run workouts even more interest and challenge.

Tempo Run

Let's start with the basics. The tempo run is a staple of the running workout calendar.

A tempo run is a great all-around run, whether you're doing 5Ks or marathons. The idea of a tempo run is to train just below your lactate threshold, or the threshold where your body switches to relying on the anaerobic energy system, specifically the lactate or glycolytic systems. Some people call this a threshold run.

A good tempo run will leave you feeling spent but not completely exhausted. It will give both your legs and your lungs a great workout, and

Runner's Magazine even claimed that the tempo run might be the single most important run to do in your repertoire.

If you want to vary this workout, experiment by pushing above your lactate or anaerobic thresholds.

Here is the idea with a tempo run. Warm up with a slow pace, and then increase your speed to a fast pace that is aout30 seconds slower than your 5K race pace, or pretty close to your marathon pace. Maintain that speed for a couple miles or more if you have the time.

It should be "comfortably hard": you should feel like you are at about 85% of all-out effort (assuming your warm-up was at about 20% effort).

Intensity: Medium

7-minute warm-up
22 minutes at pace :30 seconds off your 5K race pace
Brief cool-down

Cut-down Runs

The cut-down is another classic running workout. Simple and basic, but so effective. Ask any marathon coach, and they will tell you that a cut-down run is a regular tool in their arsenal. A cut-down run is a favorite among many longer-distance coaches, but it isn't just for long runs – the concept applies such as effectively to shorter runs.

The typical cut-down run is pretty long -- 10 miles or more if you are a marathoner -- but the concept can be applied to any run. In a short run, you can use the cut-down to help give you some workout variety without the frequent intervals of some of my other workouts.

The cut-down run works so well because it allows you to get all systems working for a sustained period of time, and work on your cadence and stride, things that are hard to do if you keep changing your pace. It is also an easy workout to do if you forgot your training watch (or are without one) especially if you know your route well and have mental markers of the various distance segments.

Below is a great cut-down run that can work for the 5K or 10K runner.

Intensity: Medium

7 min warmup (this counts as part of your first segment for the cut-down).
1 mile at 1 minute slower than your 5K pace
1 miles at 30 seconds slower than your 5K pace
½ mile at your 5K pace
3-5 minute cool down

Fartleks

Swedish for "speed play", the Fartlek is a funny-sounding workout that's incredibly effective for every skill level. Not to play favorites, but it might be the single best and simplest "rut-buster" on this entire list. The Swedes gave the running community a great workout in this one.

Simply put, a Fartlek is a combination of fast and slow running. The beauty of it is that it can be done in virtually any setting. Some runners do Fartlek intervals by timing with a watch, others based on telephone poles, and others based on intersections or other markers. If you have a GPS watch, you can use that, too.

A Fartlek can be done using a high degree of structure or very little. Here's a simple example of a Fartlek workout that anyone with a watch (or an IPod with a clock) can do.

Warm up, then time yourself to do two minutes hard, at about a hard mile pace or faster, followed by two minutes of very slow jogging. During the slow jog, don't worry about speed at all. Just keep your feet moving and let your heart rate come back down. Repeat this sequence four to ten times total, depending on your level of fitness and the race you're training for.

Using a GPS watch to keep your fast pace at a target is a great way to keep your legs honest later in this set. This type of workout will not only improve your aerobic capacity; it will also enhance your ability to recover.

Intensity: High

7-minute warm-up
2 minutes hard (mile pace or faster), followed by 2 minutes slow. Repeat 5 times.
3 minute cool-down.

Recovery Run

The recovery run is a highly-debated part of the running regimen. Many say that there is no purpose in a recovery run, you either run or you rest. Others say that, especially during the "build" and "peak" phases, recovery runs are beneficial. I side with them, the latter. I think that recovery runs are good for people, and help them stay in the cadence of working-out while allowing the runner somewhat of a day off.

A good workout run needs to be easy. The perfect workout run is a 30 minute sustained run at 60-70% of your heart rate reserve (HRR). The HRR is the difference between resting and maximum heart rates. For example, if your resting heart rate is 60, and your max heart rate is 170, your HRR is the 110 beats in between. 65% of that would be around 132 beats per minute. That is not a hard run.

A second way of looking at recovery runs is that they should always be done at conversation pace. If you are unable to carry on a normal conversation with a running mate, you are going too fast.

Besides recovering, this kind of run has a way of using your fat stores, something we all want. Lower bodyfat means a leaner running body. The recovery run is a good change of pace from all of your supercharged training runs.

Intensity: Low

30 minutes at 65% of your HRR

Simple Intervals

A form of the Fartlek, this workout gets a little more intensity with your speed and your fast-twitch work. Like the Fartlek, this is one of the simplest running workouts you can do, but also one of the most effective. The even alternation between fast running and easy recovery accumulates through the workout, and by the final 5 intervals you will begin to feel some oxygen debt happening. This type of workout will help train your heart rate to recover quickly after exertion, something that will help your overall conditioning.

Your speed during the fast intervals should be a little above your fast 5K pace. It should not be an all-out sprint (we will get to that workout next) but rather a nice, fast clip where you are quite winded by the 1-minute mark.

Exactly how hard you go will depend on your conditioning. For most people, the minute of easy running will not be enough to fully recover, so you will notice your speed to decrease and fatigue to increase by the 10th interval.

Doing this workout correctly should bring you up above the anaerobic threshold during the back part of the hard interval. As we have learned, training at or slightly above your threshold can help gradually raise the threshold, which will help you increase your overall speed and conditioning.

Intensity: High

7 min warmup
1 minute hard run followed immediately by 1 minute easy recovery jog.
Repeat 10 times.
3 min cool down

Sprint Intervals (aka speed blasts)

Sprint intervals, or speed blasts as they are often called in the running community, take intervals to the next level. During the workout, you will want to aim for a pace that is an all-out sprint. Think about how fast you might try to finish a 5K race with someone you want to beat right beside you.

The sprint is followed by 2 minutes of easy running. During this phase, don't worry about your heart rate or exertion, the goal is to get your wind back and be in good shape for the next sprint. If you are doing the sprint legs right and with the proper intensity, 2 minutes of rest will feel like it is just a bit short for complete recovery, so each progressive interval will feel harder.

Because your sprints are only for 30 seconds, you probably won't spend much time in your maximum (90%+) heart rate zone. You might touch it briefly, but it would be brief.

For this workout, be sure to stretch well and only do it on a good, safe surface. Anytime you sprint, you run the risk of injuring a joint or straining a muscle.

Intensity: High

7 min warmup
30 second sprint followed by 2 minute easy recovery jog. Repeat 8 times.
3 min cool down

Negative Ladders

Any type of ladder workout is effective because it throws a lot at you. In the same workout, you will get everything from a fast 5K pace to all-out sprints to some resting jogs.

I'm not talking about old-fashioned agility ladder workouts here, the type where you literally use quick feet to run through a ladder. Rather, the ladder concept pertains to the duration and speed of various intervals. You will have everything from 5 minutes of exertion down to 1 minute of heavy exertion -- nearly a sprint. Each interval will feature a minute of rest, during which time you should slow way down -- nearly to a walk if needed -- and just focus on dropping your heart rate and catching your breath.

This workout requires a watch or timer of some sort. Most of these workouts do, actually, but this one in particular calls for focused time management.

Intensity: High

7 min warmup
5 min hard, 10K pace
1 min easy
4 min hard, 5K pace
1 min easy
3 min hard, 5K pace plus 10%
1 min easy
2 min hard, 5K pace plus 25%

1 min easy
1 min hard, just short of a sprint
6 min cool down

3 Minute Progressives

The progressive runs are a bit of a cross between a ladder and a true interval. Like a ladder, they throw different speeds at you during the same workout. Unlike a ladder, you don't spend more time at slower speeds than at the faster speeds. And while the progressive runs use even interval times to give you a quality workout, they rotate between 3 or more different workout speeds.

In addition to being a quality cardio workout, this is a great way to work on your stride as well. Work on your stride length and refining the right kind of foot strike. Start with shorter, quick strides, and work your way into longer, graceful strides.

I like these workouts for my moderate runs, when I want a good, quality workout but would prefer to keep my heart rate in the aerobic zone for a good overall cardio workout. If you are just thinking of going for "a run", consider making it a progressive so you can add a bit of variety to it. Your body will thank you.

Intensity: Medium

6 minute warmup
1 minute easier run at brisk conversational pace
1 minute at 10K pace
1 minute at 5K pace
Repeat 7 times
3 min cool down

Running tempo – Negative Splits

This is a variation on the tempo run, and it can easily be done in any location where know the route and distances within it. This workout is designed to help improve your VO2 max and give you speed for the "kick" of a short race. It can also get you ready for the intensity of a longer race.

As an avid 5K runner, I like to plan a route that includes a nice, easy warm-up, as I do with all my runs.

If you plan your route right, the next couple miles should be in an area relatively free of pedestrians or traffic lights. I like to run the next two miles just a bit off my race pace —definitely too fast for conversation. For example, if my race pace was 7:30 minutes per mile, I would want to be at 8:00 or faster. Then, I would adjust down for mile 2, closer to race pace. For the final ½ mile, try to build up to your 5K pace.

This workout is best done during the "build" phase of your training plan. If you're a 10Ker or half marathoner, concentrate on lengthening your running stride during this run.

Intensity: Medium

7-minute warm-up
1 mile at a pace :30 seconds off your 5K pace
1 mile at a pace :15 seconds off your 5K pace
½ mile at a pace near your 5K race pace
Brief cool-down

5K Pace Bursts

A "burst" style run can be done with any distance, but knowing that this book is intended for the time-constrained athlete, I focus on shorter bursts. For the typical runner or triathlete, having some type of burst workout is great. It allows your legs and lungs to experience a bit of unpredictability, and helps you build for some moderate leg strength in cases where you are moving into your "build" or "peak" zone of periodization.

I like the burst workouts because they make what would normally be a pretty bland run into something that has some intellectual interest as well as the ability to spike up to an anaerobic level, but just for a short period of time before resting.

For runs like the Bursts, when you will be exerting yourself hard for a sustained number of minutes, you should train with a heart rate monitor. As I mentioned early in the book, some of these workouts can be pretty intense, and this is one where you want your heart rate to drift up into the hard, 80-90% range, but not higher.

Intensity: Medium/High

7 min warmup
4 minutes at fast 5K pace -- about as fast as you could ever do a 5K
2 mins rest
Repeat 4 times

Enjoying the Book?

Are you enjoying these workouts so far? I'd love to hear what you think! Consider leaving a review to let others know, as well. You can do that here.

Alactic-Aerobic Intervals

This workout offers more speed work, so you can really increase your foot speed and leg strength. A simple Alactic-Aerobic Interval is a great workout that can be done nearly anywhere: a track, a trail, a quiet street, or even a treadmill. Included in your workout routine once a week, it can give your running capacity a great boost, especially if you're a sprint triathlete or a 5Ker.

Like many of our workouts, simplicity is one of this workout's best features.

Do your warm-up and get a good stretch. Then begin a set of about 20 short sprints, all-out, each followed by about 40 seconds of rest. The sprints should be about 6 to 8 seconds long and require you to be at 100% effort. Give yourself enough rest in between to let your heart rate decrease to about 120 bpm or less. As you increase your conditioning, add more reps of sprints into the workout.

Because you don't need much space for this one – you really won't cover that much ground – this is a great workout to do if you are relegated to a park or smaller area without long trails. You can get a high-quality workout without running for miles and miles.

Intensity: Medium

7-minute warm-up
20-25 reps of 8-second sprint followed by 40-second standing or walking rest
10-minute cool-down

Out and Back, Back Hard

This workout might not seem that scientific, but does it ever work!

For anyone who has fallen into the slow pace groove, the simple out and back, with the back part being at race pace, can be a great rut-buster. This workout is especially targeted for those who might be training for a 5K, 10K, or sprint triathlon.

This kind of workout, like the Fartlek above, provides you with all-important speed work. Once you have the aerobic capacity built up from weeks or months of training, your speed is what will limit you in a shorter race. This workout will help acclimate you to a race pace.

For this kind of workout, find a good out-and-back trail with a friendly surface, such as crushed rock, gravel, or smooth asphalt. After a warm-up and a stretch, run out to a destination that's slightly farther than half of your targeted race distance. For a 5K runner, each half would be 2.5K, so find a route that will take you out 3K and back 3K.

Going out, run at a nice, slow stride, well under your race pace. At the turn, take a one-minute breather, stretch again if needed, and drink some water. Then, turn around and run at race pace or higher back to your origination point.

This type of workout will give you the feel of a race with minimal risk of overtraining, since the fast part covers a shorter distance. More importantly, it will inject much-needed variety into your running week.

Intensity: High

7-minute warmup (in the direction you plan to run back from)
Run at moderate pace, 12 or so minutes, to the turnaround point.
Turn around, and run back at fast race pace, all-out
Use any spare time for a cool-down

Section 2:
Treadmill Workouts

Treadmill workouts can be similarly precise. While running inside is often seen as a necessary evil, when you are moved indoors for your workouts, you have the ability to be carefully-measured in your speed, intervals, and exertion level.

4-Pronged Ladders

Sometimes you need a good treadmill workout, but one that is more than just a simple progression of speed. Most runners, on a treadmill, either run at the same speed the entire time or gradually increase their speed throughout the run. Both are better than nothing, but here is a better workout.

Because you can so easily manage your speed on a treadmill, this type of 4-pronged ladder works well. After your warmup, you start thinking about 2-minute segments. The first is a jog -- about 2 minutes slower than your 5K pace. Then, increase by 1mph for the next segment, which will have you moving at a good run. Then, do 2 minutes at your 5K pace, which for most people will be a few ticks faster than the last segment. Finally, finish it off with 30 seconds a little faster, as fast as you can *safely* do on a treadmill.

Cycle through that three times, and you will give your legs a nice jolt and a good workout.

For safety reasons, never run as fast on a treadmill as you would on a safe, flat, outdoor path. Always stay in control on a treadmill.

Intensity: High

7 min warmup
2 minute jog
2 minute run - 1mph above warmup speed
2 minute fast run - 5K pace
30 sec - safe sprint
Repeat 3 times.
3 min cool down

Treadmill Fartleks

Sometimes you have no choice but to run indoors, on a treadmill. Maybe it's pouring rain outside, or maybe it's the middle of winter and you don't want to risk running on ice and having that split-second accident that would result in months of rehab.

When relegated to a treadmill, you don't have to give up on the inspiring workouts. In many ways, the treadmill can be a useful change of pace, because you can completely control every aspect of your speed and incline. That gives you precise control over the intensity of your training.

I like to begin with a 7-minute warm-up run, getting the legs moving and making sure your stride is used to the slightly adapted gait of a treadmill. Once you have completed that, move on to a series of fartleks that are carefully managed by the timer on your machine.

Some treadmills will allow you to program the intervals; on others, it will be simpler to manage them manually.

Aim for two minutes of faster running followed by two minutes of recovery, for about five to ten reps (20 to 40 minutes) total, depending on your level of fitness. I like the faster intervals to be at about my race pace, or perhaps just a bit slower.

Keep in mind that on a treadmill, you're fighting the machine in addition to the motion of your body. There's no point in going all-out and injuring yourself. Keep it controlled, and you'll get an excellent indoor workout. Finish with five to ten minutes of cool-down.

Intensity: High

7-minute easy warm-up.
5 reps of 2 minutes fast (5K pace) and 2 minutes slower (1:30 off your 5K pace) for 20-minute total set.
Finish with short cool-down.

Short hill repeats

One of my favorite running workouts, especially when short on time, is to find a hill and do repeats. This is easier said than done in some parts of the country, but even a bridge or river valley can provide plenty of elevation to provide an adequate hill workout.

This kind of workout directly translates to leg strength and muscle-building, something that you don't' get as much of on your longer, flatter runs.

Start by finding a hill that provides good grade for at least 50 meters. A little longer is better, but 50 will do if you're in a flat area. The goal is to find a hill that's challenging to run and leaves you fatigued by the end but isn't so difficult that you can't complete it without slowing down to a jog or walk.

Depending on your level of fitness, you'll want to do anywhere from five to twelve reps, all with a maximal level of exertion. Run down the hills at a slow jog – there's no benefit from running downhill fast – and repeat.

Don't give yourself too much rest. You should be progressively more fatigued as you begin each rep, but do give your heart rate a chance to recover moderately between runs.

This type of workout will improve your running speed and power, as well as your lactate use and recovery.

Intensity: High

7-minute warmup
Do 5 to 12 hill repeats, hard. Exact number depends on length of hill.
Leave enough time for a 3-5 minute cool-down run.

Finish at race pace

We love adding one small twist to a nice, long run to add intensity. By doing the last half-mile or mile at race pace, you can really add some value to an otherwise routine run that might be causing a rut for you.

The best type of run for a "race pace finish" is a nice, moderate-distance run on a familiar trail. The familiarity of the route creates a dynamic where you can mentally and physically build up to the final kick because you know the route distances well.

When you hit the "one mile to go" mark, increase from your moderate pace to something at or even slightly above your race pace. This type of workout resembles a lactate threshold workout. It can do wonders to make you faster and more efficient at race pace.

If you do this, be sure you stretch before and after, as any muscle imbalances are often exacerbated during a hard kick.

Intensity: Medium

7 minute warmup
2 miles at moderately-fast clip, about 75% of max speed
Final ½ to 1 mile (depending on time remaining) at 5K race pace or slightly higher

Section 3:
Track Workouts

For any runner, <u>finding a track</u> is valuable activity and opens up a world of new and different workouts to consider. For many, the track workouts can add a certain precision to the training, as well as speed work. Doing high-intensity, short-burst (or medium-burst) speed work can help you build leg strength and feel what it is like to really get your heart rate up.

Track Workout #1: Martin and Coe

Martin and Coe wrote the book on distance running training. In doing so, they combined medical research with performance coaching. One of their favorite workouts combines shorter speed training with longer runs at race pace or above.

This is an adaptation of that workout, to help it fit into a 30-minute window.

Done correctly and with full effort, this type of workout will give your body a different training stimulus than it is used to. Done weekly, this workout will no doubt make you faster, and it can help break you out of whatever rut you might be in.

After a warm-up, the heavy training of the day will begin with two 200-meter runs, at a sprint or near-sprint. For the 200s, you should be well above your lactate threshold. Then, you will move to the longer distance work, doing a 1,000-meter run at a pace just a bit faster than 5K pace.

Once you finish the 1K, you should be pretty tired, but you're not done. Next, repeat the two200's, just like you did at the beginning of the workout.

This workout is intended for 5K specialists, but you can adjust it to meet your needs. The best place to adjust is by lengthening the 1Ks in the middle. The 200s are important for your speed and anaerobic power, regardless of what distance you run on race day.

Intensity: High

7-minute warm-up
2 x 200 meters at near-sprint, 45 seconds rest in-between
1 x 1,000 meters at better than your 5K pace,
2 x 200 meters at near-sprint, 45-seconds in-between

Track Workout #2: Keep It Simple

The beauty of a track workout is that you can keep it incredibly simple. This workout is about as simple as you can get, but very effective. For this workout, you simply run the race distance you normally do, at a speed at or above your race day speed. However, you will take short breaks throughout the run.

For a 5K runner, start with a warm-up of 7 minutes. Next, do a 1K at or above your race pace. (30 seconds/mile faster than race day is a good training pace and will improve your racing speed.) For most updated tracks, a 1K will be exactly two and a half laps around.

Follow that with 60 seconds of rest, and then repeat two more times. This workout is simple and basic, but it will help kick your running into a higher

---

gear. Doing this once a week will improve your pace on race day. It will also improve your lactate threshold.

Intensity: High

7-minute warm-up
3 x 1K at 30 seconds faster than 5K pace. 60 seconds standing rest in between.
4-8 minute cool-down

Track Workout Mid-Speed (400s)

When you head to the track, you want to take advantage of the venue to do some good speedwork. If all you are doing is a long, slow distance or recovery run, there is no point in being at a track.

I like the track for some good mid-distance speed work. There is something about the visual of knowing where I am on a track that causes me to dig a little deeper during the 2nd half of any hard interval.

One of my favorite workouts focuses on the middle-distance speed, with 400s. From the days I was a high school track runner, I have long considered the 400 one of the most difficult distances to run hard. It is too short to settle in to a comfortable pace, but too long to be able to sprint the entire way. It is a distance that will quickly tell you what kind of shape you are in. Putting your body under the stress of a fast 400 meter run will translate to your ability to attack hills or accelerate mid-race, come race-day.

This workout is one that I adapted from a running coach I once worked with, who liked to keep things simple. You will do 8 by 400 meters, at a pace that pushes you to the max but is perhaps just a few seconds short of all-out. Why? Because you only get 30 seconds of rest and then you will go again.

Expect your final 400s to be markedly slower than your first ones. This workout will wear you out.

Intensity: High

7 minute warmup
400 meter run -- very hard, but just shy of full speed. 30 seconds standing rest after each 400.
Repeat 7 times
6 minute cool down

Section 4:
Creative Run Workouts

Sometimes the best run is one that takes you to a different place, or helps you inject a different type of running altogether – finding steps, a trail for a true "trail run," or other different type of run setting can really recharge your batteries.

Find a Trail

This workout isn't so much a training plan as it is a suggestion to try something different. I love finding a trail for a good, old-fashioned trail run. My requirements are few: It needs to be in an area where the terrain will be unpredictable -- lots of up-and-down is good. Conditions need to be favorable do I don't hurt myself. And I want this type of run to be in an area of visual interest, so the workout goes by quickly.

A trail run, in the true sense, is on a trail through the woods or another rugged area. Think of what kind of trails singletrack bikers like to ride on. It should be winding, have lots of up-and-down, and be an area where you need to keep your eyes on the ground at all times. This is not a run on the paved trail that goes through your local park.

Why do I like these runs? Because they allow you to combine your brain function -- the need to constantly read the ground ahead of you and adjust accordingly -- with your cardio function. Such a run typically goes by surprisingly fast.

You just need to be extra-sure that you keep yourself healthy and safe. Trail runs can be real ankle-twisters. Never do a trail run in low-light, watch the ground at all times, and consider ditching the music for this one. Stay safe. If you do, a trail run can be an excellent - and fun - addition to your cross-training.

Steps

Rocky. If you are over 40, or have an interest in classic movies, you know the scene. Rocky runs up the steps at the Philadelphia Museum of Art, to the tune of Eye of the Tiger in the background. Most people think of that iconic scene when I tell them to run steps.

For most of us, running steps isn't nearly as iconic, but it is still a quality workout. Running steps can be a great way to cross-train your legs and lungs, and help you prepare for elevation that might require shorter, faster steps. It hardwires the need to shorten your stride when on any type of uphill climb.

Find at least 30 steps in one place. In some areas, the steps might be built-in to the side of a public area of a hill or mountain. In flatter areas, you might need to find a stadium.

They key to running steps is simple. It is in knowing that **the benefit of running steps is in the incline, not the decline**. There is literally no benefit of running down steps, and in fact there is a good chance you can hurt your joints when you do it.

If you do steps, I suggest a flat, 7-minute warmup run. Then, do sets of sprints up the steps until you hit the 25-minute mark of your workout, and finish by doing a 5-minute cool-down. The key is that when you sprint up the steps, stop at the top and then walk back down. You can walk somewhat quickly, but don't run. Running downhill has few if any benefits.

Intensity: Medium

7-minute warmup
Run up at a steady, quick pace, and walk down. Repeat for 18 minutes.
5-minute cool-down

Running – Destination run

Sometimes it's not changing the intensity or the mileage that you need, but rather mixing up the venue.

I was once in a rut where every workout I did was a four-mile run on the exact same cinder trail. I was maintaining my fitness, but I wasn't breaking through to the next level. The solution was to drive to a small river island that had a trail around the outside of it.

A change in venue, including different terrain as well as scenery, can leave you with a better workout and begin the process of breaking through that plateau.

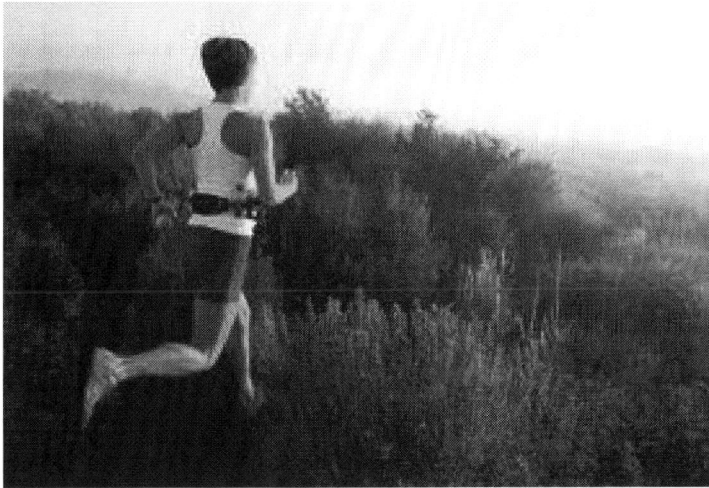

If you're a member of a local running club, you should have access to many different venues. Most running clubs post route options on their websites or have a forum where runners can compare various routes.

You can also simply get a map and look for regional or state parks, which usually have great scenery and some type of trail network.

Finally, there are some online resources that can map your run. These are great if you are looking for a new route, but something in an area you already have in mind. MapMyRun might be my favorite at the moment.

Do a 5K

There's nothing like an actual race to make you run at a faster pace or with a higher intensity level. You can do as many race simulations as you want, but until you hear a starting gun and run among others at your target pace, you will never quite be able to dig in and find that elusive extra gear.

Signing up for a local 5K can be an incredible way to take your training to the next level. It pushes you to a higher intensity level than you would do on your own, and it takes away the comfort of being on your normal running trail or starting the run on your own schedule. The addition of other racers is an intangible that is very difficult, if not impossible, to replicate.

The best part about 5Ks is that in most metro areas or mid-sized towns, you can find a 5K nearly every weekend of the summer and fall. I suggest *not* doing a large, well-known, but rather a smaller neighborhood 5K. They are simpler, the crowds or fewer, and the arrival and departure is made much easier.

Section 5:
Cross Training

Cross training belongs in every athlete's training plan. Effective cross-training helps balance your workouts and prevent injury by reducing overuse injuries. It also has huge benefits on your overall strength and coordination. The age-old Muscle Confusion Principle suggests that your muscles tend to accommodate the exercise they are used to, and by stressing them in new ways, you will grow.

The cross-training I suggest ranges from mixing HIIT into your runs, to doing completely different activities – swimming is a favorite.

20 Minute Moderate Run + HIIT

One paradox of run training is that sometimes you feel best when you are doing more than just running. In fact, one thing I try to do anytime I have the time for it is incorporate some HIIT to the end of a run. I have a 5-minute "flow" that I often tack on to the end of a run, and variations of that flow are easy to tack on regardless of how much time I have to spare.

I write about the importance of adding core, yoga, or HIIT work to your run training in one of my other books, _Running Smarter_.

I will share with you a great circuit that you can tack-on to the end of any run. It will leave you feeling like you gave your core and upper body some work, in addition to your legs. It is best to do this after a not-so-hard run, because if you really wear yourself out on a run, the odds are that your form for any core work will be poor due to fatigue.

The circuit is a simple 10-minute workout, followed by 2 cycles of exercises. You start with mountain climbers, in the plank position but quickly pulling your knees to your chest four times, followed by a pushup. Repeat for a minute. Then, you do vertical jumps. In a controlled way, try to explode straight up with a vertical jump, ensuring that you are really engaging your hip thrust. Then, do a minute of plank, however you prefer -- arms, elbows, side. Then, a minute of half burpees -- the kind with no pushup. Then rest for a minute, and do it all one more time.

I recommend doing this after an easy, 20 minute run. It can be a great recovery workout to flush out your muscles and give you some cross-training.

Intensity: Medium

Run 20 minutes, conversation pace.

10-minute Circuit
1 min mountain climbers w/ pushup
1 minute vertical jumps
1 minute plank
1 minute ½ burpees
1 minute rest
Repeat the cycle one more time for 10 minutes of total circuit work

Run and Plyo

The run and plyo workout is a riff on the circuit workout, above. Instead of doing the circuit or HIIT work at the end, you do it during the run. This can be a great cross-training option for those days when you want to be outside, but your training plan doesn't call for hard mileage. It can also be great for those times when your body is telling you it needs a more balanced training day.

Because stopping for 2 minutes will drop your heart rate (with the exception of the burpees, which may actually increase it), I suggest doing the run legs at a pretty good clip -- around a 10K pace -- in order to stay in your heart rate training zone.

You will see some of the same exercises in this workout as in my other HIIT workout, because I love mountain climbers, burpees, and plank. They work so many muscle groups at the same time, and they all work your core.

This workout includes 8 minute runs at a moderately fast pace, interspersed with 2 minutes of plyo or core work. You do three 10-minute cycles of that, and then you are done.

Intensity: Medium

8 minute run at warmup pace
1 minute mountain climbers, 1 minute of plank
8 minute run at 10K pace
1 minute of burpees, 1 minute of side plank
8 minute run at 10K pace
1 minute of jumping jacks, 1 minute of bicycle crunches

Mini Bricks

A brick workout is one of the iconic triathlon-specific workouts, and it benefits you even if you are not a triathlete. The level of cross-training that you get in a brick is an excellent change-up for your legs, and your cardiovascular system.

Mini-bricks take the brick concept a step farther, giving your body multiple exercise stimuli and creating excellent range in your fitness and lactate thresholds.

Mini-bricks are similar to bricks except the sets are shorter, and there are more of them. Instead of doing one bike ride followed by one run, a good mini-brick workout may have 3 sets of the activities.

Even better, they're a great workout to try when you're relegated to a health club session, such as on a rainy or icy day. My favorite mini-bricks are about 45 minutes long, and simply have 10 minutes of riding followed by 5 minutes of running, repeated three times. You can adjust the distances based on your fitness level and desired race distance.

Like the bricks above, the mini-bricks will improve your workout capacity and exercise economy.

Intensity Level: Medium

7-minute running warm-up
8 minutes hard cycling immediately followed by a 4-minute run, with no rest in between sets. Repeat two times.

Cycling – Spinning with an online stream, app, or DVD

Many cyclists abhor indoor trainers. (An indoor trainer is a device that you prop your bike on to work out indoors during bad weather.) But it is gaining significant popularity, due to everything from the need to get off the roads and away from traffic, to the advent of the smart trainer – an incredible device that allows you high-quality spin workouts at home. The smart trainer is a gamechanger!

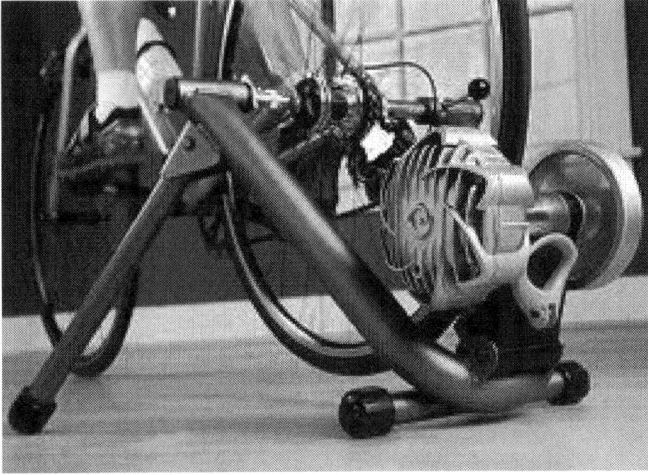

Truth be told, trainers can provide some great cycling workouts as well as much-needed training progressions, so we recommend integrating them into your workout. We highly recommend the Spinervals line of workouts or an app like Zwift or Sufferfest, but there are others on the market as well. All have a variety of specific workouts that can give you different total workout durations and intensity levels. These workouts allow you to focus on technique at various power outputs.

Using a trainer with a structured workout has many benefits. One benefit is the ability to build leg speed and work on your power output within a periodized program. More importantly, indoor cycling allows you to manage your lactate threshold and manipulate your heart rate precisely. These are difficult to do when you're riding outside on varied terrain and being interrupted by stoplights and traffic.

Cycling – Lactate Threshold Time Trial

Without getting into too much detail, the Lactate Threshold (LT) is the point during a workout when lactate builds up in your blood faster than your body can remove it. The LT can also be explained as the level of intensity in which the body switches from using the aerobic system to using the anaerobic system as its major energy supply. In layman's terms, it's the point during a hard workout at which you build fatigue and begin to lose power. Increasing this threshold allows you to maintain a higher power output during a race or difficult workout.

There are several ways to measure your LT. The simplest is to use a heart rate monitor during a very hard, 30-minute workout. Your average heart rate over that very hard workout is your LT.

Once you know your LT, you can build in training at or just above your LT for a period of 20-30 minutes. A great way to improve your lactate threshold is to mix in an LT-focused worked about once a week.

Increasing your LT uses a process very similar to measuring it: training more frequently around the threshold will cause it to increase.

Intensity: High

7 minute warm-up ride
20 minutes very hard riding, with a heart rate monitor measuring at 100% - 105% of your LT.
Brief cool-down

Swimming – 1 hard by 3 easy

I was never a swimmer growing up, but I started doing occasional swims as I trained for triathlons. An amazing thing happened – the swimming made my running lung capacity much better.

For a new swimmer, just getting in the pool will be a workout in itself. When you need to inject some intensity into your swim workout, the main way to do it is to add speed and effort at various parts of the session. Here's one way to create speed that can be done in any pool and under nearly any conditions. It simply adds a hard, all-out lap or pool-length in a group of four, giving you a nice 1x3 sequence.

This is as simple as it sounds. Before you start, warm up with whatever sequence you prefer. Once you're warmed up, simply swim one pool length as hard as you can, well above your lactate threshold. You should be winded at the end, especially as you get deeper into the workout. Then, recover with three pool lengths of easy or moderate swimming.

Repeat this sequence as many times as needed to get your desired total workout time, when factoring in a cool-down. An alternative for more advanced swimmers is to replace a pool-length with a full lap, doubling the rep length.

Intensity: Medium

Warm up for 7 minutes or your typical warmup duration
Swim 12-20 minutes, repeating 1 pool length very hard followed by 3 lengths moderate. Cool down for 3-8 minutes.

Swimming – Fast Ladder

Ladders, or pyramids, are great workouts for all types of activities. They're often overlooked in swimming.

Let's say you're trying to improve your lung capacity, or maybe you are even a triathlete training for a Sprint race, and your swim training consists of swimming a moderate 800 to 1000 meters twice a week. This is better than nothing, but it's conducive to entering the dreaded rut. A simple ladder can add some variety and intensity to your swim workout, without adding total training time to your calendar.

In swimming, a ladder focuses hitting near-maximal effort for a portion in the middle of your swim workout. During this hard effort, your heart rate should increase considerably, and you should feel your arm, shoulder, and leg muscles working overtime.

This style of workout is called a ladder because you might start with 100 meters hard, then 150 meters, then 200 meters, then perhaps 250, all with some slow recovery in between.

This workout can break you out of your rut. Add a good warm-up and cool-down, and you'll have yourself a nice 30 minute workout.

Intensity: Medium

7 minutes of warm-up
100 meters hard, 50 easy
150 meters hard, 50 easy
200 meters hard, 50 easy
100 meters hard, remainder of time easy

Summary

Runners from 5K'ers to ultra-marathoners benefit from a variety of challenging workouts, and I know from experience that having some time-saving workouts can be a huge benefit for your training schedule.

I hope you enjoy these workouts, and I hope they allow you to break out of the rut with your training. If you use this book the way I hope you will, it will become a reference for years to come, rather than a book that you read once and put on the shelf.

It would mean a lot to me if you considered leaving a review for this book. You can do that here.

If you enjoyed this, consider checking out my other work.

Your First Triathlon Guide - My top-selling book, helping people around the world enter the sport of triathlon. Triathlon is a great way to experience balanced fitness.

Running Smarter - 21 workout and nutrition "hacks' to help you become a more capable runner, regardless of your goals.

Fit Foods - A guide on how athletes can use everyday nutrition to their advantage, in a way that is actionable and sustainable.

If you want to hear about **the best running tips and gear deals I am finding**, feel free sign up for my mailing list. I only email when there is something valuable for you. Don't worry, you will never get spammed. Sign up here.

Resources

The following resources are useful to runners, swimmers, triathletes and cyclists as you focus on reaching new milestones.

Your First Triathlon Guide: Do a Triathlon in 100 Days or Less. Our guide to getting in shape for your first triathlon, and a practical step-by-step tutorial for new triathletes.

Triathlon Wetsuit Store. An online resource devoted to triathlon training tips and gear, but useful to any swimmer, runner, or cyclist. Offers many discounts on high quality workout gear.

Total Immersion Swim Training. The best swim technique training on the market, and an avid marketer of instructional DVDs. Use the code "TWSTI" for discounts at checkout.

Xterra. Makers of top-of-the-line workout gear and wetsuits. Use the code "EBOOK" for major discounts at checkout.

Printed in Great Britain
by Amazon